Your Free Gift

I wanted to show my appreciation that you support my work so I've put together a free gift for you.

Slowcooker Essentials Cookbook

http://thezenfactory.com/mediterranean_-diet-_free_book/

Just visit the link above to download it now.

I know you will love this gift.

Thanks!

Table of Contents

Introduction

The Mediterranean Diet is not just a diet, it is a way of life that everyone should follow. The delicious flavors of the Mediterranean cannot be beat, especially when you are looking to live a healthier life.

The Mediterranean Diet focuses on lean meats, healthy fats and the consumption of plenty of vegetables. You have the ability to enjoy more food while consuming less calories than the average diet.

You will love all 51 of these delicious recipes and you will love this book from beginning to end. Our ingredients lists make it easy to make your grocery list and even easier to put your meals together.

We have used easy to follow directions so that you do not have to worry about the time it will take for you to cook your meals.

Live Longer By Eating the Mediterranean Diet

The ancient Mediterranean civilization is full of stories and historic events. The Mediterranean civilization is one of the most distinguished ancient civilizations and it has influenced a multitude of other cultures around the world. Because of the geographical location of the Mediterranean, it had the ability to influence a great deal of other civilizations.

After many years, the Mediterranean diet took hold of the Western World. Now that science has improved, it has been proven that for centuries the people of the Mediterranean had the perfect idea. The diet that they have followed for centuries that is rich in olive oil is nutritionally sound. It has also been proven that by following the diet have a lower risk of heart disease and obesity.

In contrast to the American diet, the Mediterranean diet includes mostly fresh, seasonal vegetables, low to moderate amounts of dairy, fish and poultry, only small amounts of red meat, eggs, wine and beer.

This diet contains a pretty high amount of fat to be so healthy, however it is the types of fat that the diet consists of that makes it so much different. The Mediterranean diet consists of healthy fats like olive oil and omega-3 oils. The diet does not contain fried foods at all, which completely eliminates saturated fats.

The researchers from the University of Athens and the Harvard School of Public Health has recorded the dietary habits of 22,000 Greek people and found that they were much less likely to suffer from heart disease or cancer.

Even if you do not live in the Mediterranean, you can still enjoy the delicious flavors wherever you are.

Do You Love Food?

If you love food with rich flavors and bold spices, the Mediterranean is where you were meant to be. This diet is not only healthy for you, but it is simply delicious! The mix of fresh flavors will have you hooked in no time and will have you coming back for more.

There are a lot of reasons that the Mediterranean diet should rope you in. Not only does it provide bold, fresh flavors, but it also provides amazing textures and vibrant colors. Your health will thank you as well because your will be less prone to diseases both now and in the future.

A True Family Diet

The Mediterranean diet is a diet that your entire family can follow without hesitation. Your children will be healthier as well. Your kids will have the ability to try foods that they typically would never come across in American cuisine which puts them at an advantage when it comes to trying new foods. It will allow your children to develop more of an open mind when it comes to food and make them less likely to reject a food on site.

This is one diet that you do not have to feel guilty for having all of your family follow one specific diet. It will not only help them to develop better health, but it will also help them to perform better on a mental level due to all of the omega-3 fatty acids.

If you are looking for a diet with a lot of perks and very few drawbacks, you have found exactly what you are looking for. To top off all of these benefits, you don't have to feel guilty about having a glass of wine in the evening anymore!

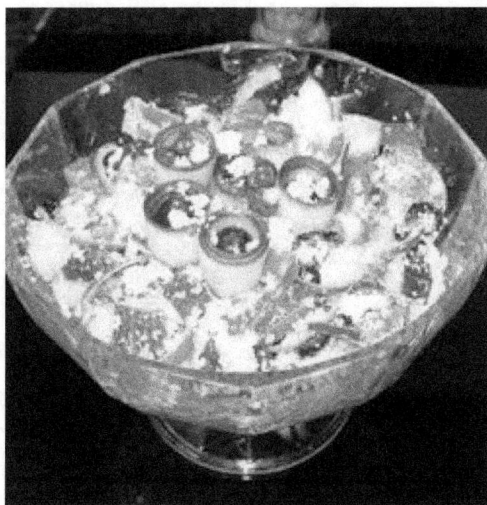

Greek Mediterranean salad

(ready in about10 minutes | Servings 1)

Ingredients:

- 1 ½ C.s – Feta cheese, crumbled
- 3 – Cucumbers, seeded and sliced
- 3 C.s – Roma tomatoes, diced
- 1 C. – Black olives, pitted and sliced
- ½ - Red onion, sliced
- 1/3 C. – Oil packed sun-dried tomatoes, diced, drained and oil reserved

Directions:

1. Toss the feta cheese, cucumbers, Roma tomatoes, olives, sun-dried tomatoes, 2 tbsps. Sun-dried reserved tomato oil, and red onion. Place the salad in the refrigerator to chill.

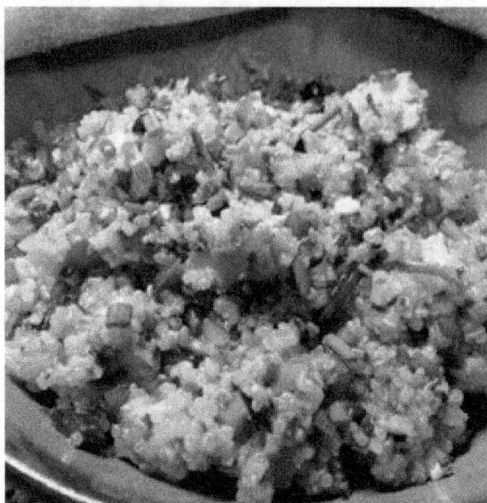

Mediterranean Quinoa Salad
(ready in about 35 minutes | Serving 4)

Ingredients:
- 2 Cubes – Chicken bouillon
- 2 C. – Water
- 1 C. – uncooked quinoa
- 1 clove – Garlic, smashed
- 1 Large – Red Onion, diced
- 2 large – Chicken breasts, cooked and cut into bite sized pieces
- ½ C. – Kalamata olives, chopped
- 1 Large – Green bell pepper, diced
- ¼ C. – Fresh parsley, chopped
- ½ C. – Feta cheese, crumbled
- ½ Tsp. – Salt
- ¼ C. – Fresh Chives, chopped
- 1 tbsp. – Balsamic Vinegar
- 2/3 C. – Lemon juice, fresh

- ¼ C. – Olive oil

Directions:

1. Place the garlic, and bouillon cubes in a saucepan with the water and bring to a boil. Stir the quinoa in and cover while lowering the heat to a medium-low. Simmer the mixture until the quinoa becomes tender and water is absorbed. This should take about 15 to 20 minutes. Place the Quinoa in a large bowl discarding the garlic clove.
2. Stir the onion, chicken, olives, bell pepper, parsley, feta cheese, salt, and chives in with the quinoa. Drizzle the top with balsamic vinegar, lemon, and olive oil. Mix it all together evenly and serve cool or warm.

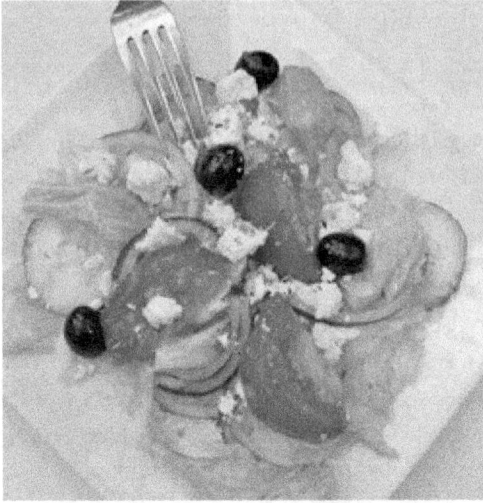

The Healthy Greek Salad
(ready in about 15 minutes | Servings 6)

Ingredients:

- 2 – Cucumbers, peeled and chopped
- 3 Large- Ripe tomatoes, chopped
- ¼ C. – Olive Oil
- 1 Small –Red onion, chopped
- 1 ½ Tsps. – Dried oregano
- 4 Tsps. – Lemon juice
- 1 C. – Feta cheese, crumbled
- Salt and Pepper
- 6 – Black Greek olives, pitted and sliced

Directions:

1. Combine cucumber, tomatoes, and onion in a salad bowl. Sprinkle with lemon juice, oil, salt and pepper, and oregano. Sprinkle olives, and feta cheese over the salad.

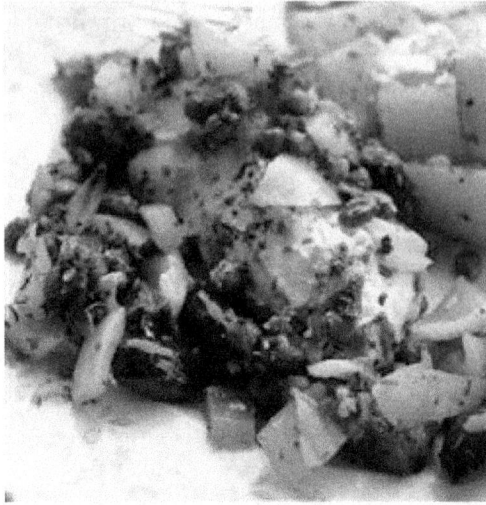

Simple Mediterranean Fish
(ready in about 45 minutes | Servings 4)

Ingredients:

- 1 Tbsp. – Greek Seasoning
- 4 (6 oz.) – Halibut fillets
- 1 – Onion, chopped
- 1 Large – Tomato, chopped
- ¼ C. – Capers
- 1 (5 oz.) – Jar Kalamata olives, pitted
- 1 Tbsp. – Lemon juice
- ¼ C. – Olive oil
- Salt and pepper

Directions:
1. Preheat your oven to 350 °F

2. Lay the halibut fillets out on a large sheet of aluminum foil. Season with your Greek seasoning. Combine onion, tomato, capers, olives, lemon juice, olive oil, pepper, and salt in a bowl. Spoon your tomato mixture over the halibut. Fold over the aluminum foil and fold the edges creating a large cooking pouch. Place the cooking pouch on a baking sheet.
3. Place in the oven to bake for 30 to 40 minutes until the fish becomes flakey.

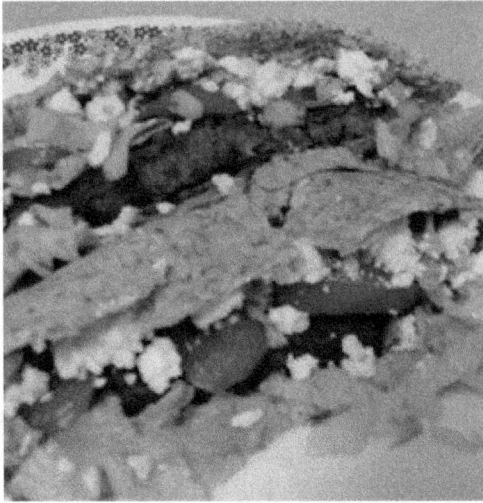

Falafel

(ready in about 55 minutes | Servings 2)

Ingredients:

- 1 can (15 oz.) – Garbanzo beans, rinsed and drained
- ¼ C. – Onion, chopped
- 3 Cloves – Garlic, minced
- ¼ C. – Fresh Parsley, chopped
- ¼ Tsp. – Ground coriander
- 1 Tsp. – Ground cumin
- ¼ Tsp. – Baking soda
- ¼ Tsp. – Salt
- 1 – Egg, beaten
- 1 Tbsp. – All-purpose flour
- 2 Tsps. – Olive oil

Directions:

1. Take your onion and wrap it in the cheese cloth, squeezing out all the moisture as possible and setting it to the side. Take your food processor and place your parsley, garbanzo beans, cumin, garlic, salt, coriander, and baking soda inside of it. Process your mixture until you have a course puree. Mix in your onion into the garbanzo bean mixture. Now stir in your egg, and flour until you have your dough and shape it into four patties letting them stand for about 15 minutes.
2. Preheat your oven to 400 °F
3. In a large pan heat your olive oil on medium-high. Place your four patties into the skillet and cook until they reach a golden brown. This should take about 3 minutes for each side.
4. Transfer the patties to your now preheated oven and bake for 10 minutes, until heated through.

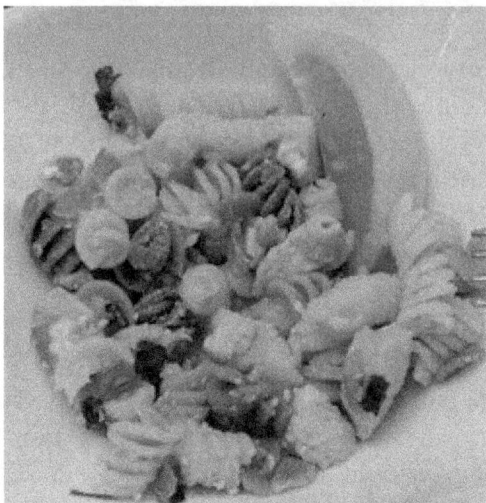

Greek Chicken Pasta

(ready in about 30 minutes | Serving 6)

Ingredients:

- ½ C. – Red onion, chopped
- 1 Pack (16 oz.) – linguine pasta
- 2 Cloves – Garlic, crushed
- 1 Tbsp. – Olive oil
- 1 Can (14 oz.) – Marinated artichoke hearts, drained and chopped
- 1 Lbs. Boneless chicken breast meat, skinless, cut into bite-size pieces
- ½ C. – Feta cheese, crumbled
- 1 Large – Tomato, chopped
- 2 Tbsps. – Lemon juice
- 3 Tbsps. – Fresh parsley, chopped
- Salt and pepper to taste
- 2 Tsps. – Dried oregano

- 2 – Lemons, wedged for garnish

Directions:

1. Using a large pot, bring salted water to a boil. Cook pasta for 8 to 10 minutes or until it is tender but still maintains a light firmness. Drain pasta and set to the side.
2. In a large skillet over medium heat, heat olive oil. Add the onion and garlic. Sauté until the mixture becomes aromatic. This should take approximately 2 minutes.
3. Stir in the chicken and cook until the juices run clear. This should take about 5 to 6 minutes.
4. Reduce the heat to medium low. Add in artichoke hearts, tomato, feta cheese, parsley, lemon juice, oregano and the pasta. Cook for an additional 3 minutes.
5. Remove the mixture from the heat and season to taste with salt and pepper.
6. Garnish with lemon wedges and serve.

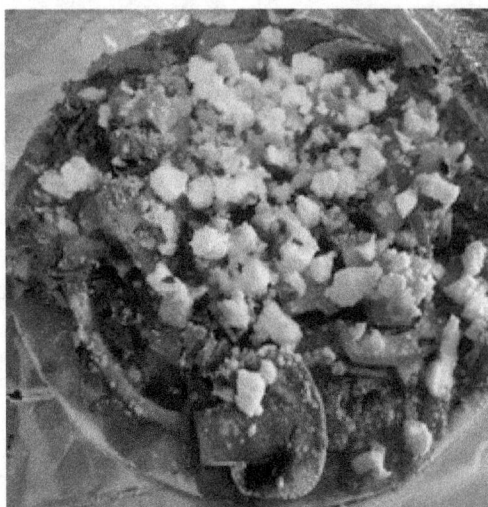

Spinach and Feta Pita Bake
(ready in about 22 minutes | Serving 6)

Ingredients:

- 3 tbsp. olive oil
- 2 tbsp. parmesan cheese, grated
- 1 (6 oz.) tub sun dried tomato pesto
- 2 tomatoes, chopped
- 4 fresh mushrooms, sliced
- 1 bunch spinach, rinsed and chopped
- ½ c. crumbled feta cheese
- 6 – 6 inch whole wheat peat bread
- Freshly ground black pepper, to taste

Directions:
1. Preheat oven to 350 degrees F.

2. Spread the pesto onto one side of each pita, like you would sauce a pizza. Place each pita on a baking sheet. Top each pita evenly with other ingredients.
3. Bake for 12 minutes. Allow pitas to cool slightly and then quarter them using a pizza cutter.
4. Serve.

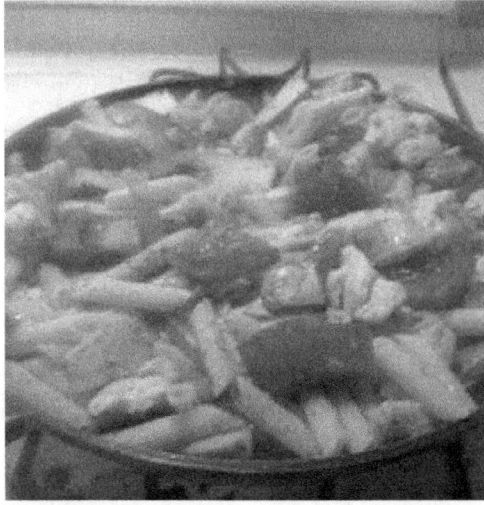

Greek Penne and Chicken
(ready in about 50 minutes | Serving 4)

Ingredients:

- 1 lb. package penne pasta
- ½ c. red onion, chopped
- 1 lb. skinless, boneless chicken breasts, sliced into bite sized pieces
- ½ c. feta cheese, crumbled
- 1 ½ tbsp. butter
- 2 large cloves garlic, minced
- 1 can (14 oz.) artichoke hearts, packed in water
- 1 large tomato, chopped
- 3 tbsp., fresh parsley, chopped
- 2 tbsp. freshly squeezed lemon juice
- 1 tsp dry oregano
- Sea salt, to taste
- Freshly ground pepper, to taste

Directions:

1. Using a large pot, bring lightly salted water to a boil. Cook pasta until it is fork-tender.
2. While pasta is cooking, heat a large skillet over medium-high heat. Melt butter. Add onion and garlic to the pan. Allow to cook for 2 minutes. Add in chicken and cook until the chicken is golden brown and juices run clear.
3. Reduce heat to medium-low.
4. Drain the artichoke hearts and chop into small pieces. Add to the pan. Add in tomatoes, feta, parsley, lemon juice, oregano and pasta. Cook the mixture together for about 3 minutes.
5. Season the mixture with salt and pepper to taste. Serve while warm.

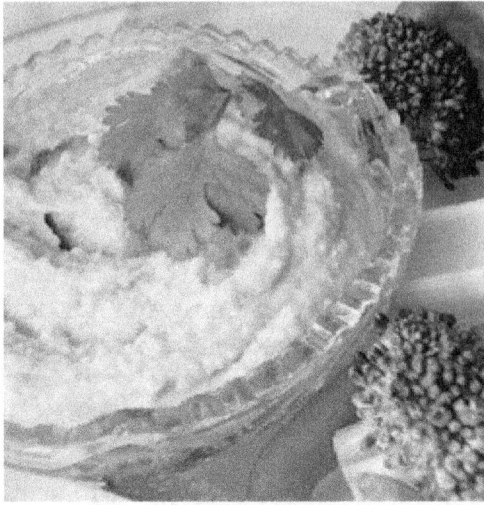

Super Easy Humus

(ready in about 5minutes | Serving 4)

Ingredients:

- 1 can (15 oz.) garbanzo beans, drained completely and liquid reserved
- 1 large clove of garlic, crushed and peeled
- 2 tsp ground cumin
- ½ tsp sea salt
- 1 tbsp. extra virgin olive oil

Directions:

1. In a blender, mix all ingredients except for the reserved garbanzo bean juice.

2. Blend the mixture on low speed, gradually adding the garbanzo bean liquid until the humus has reached the desired consistency.
3. Serve.

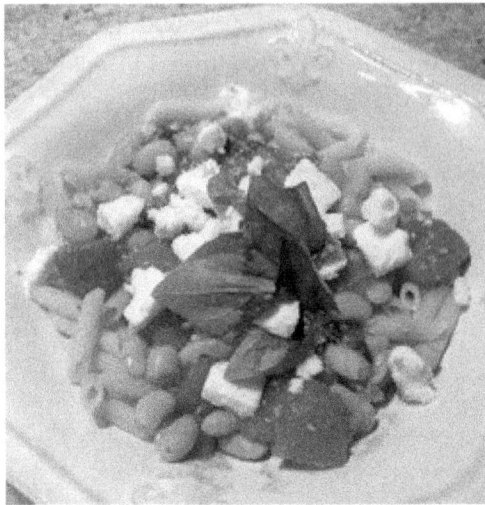

Greek Pasta with Tomatoes and White Beans

(ready in about 25 minutes | Serving 4)

Ingredients:

- 2 cans (14.5 oz. each) Italian-style diced tomatoes
- 1 (19 oz.) can cannellini beans, thoroughly drained and rinsed well
- 10 oz. fresh spinach, washed, dried and chopped
- 8 oz. penne pasta
- ½ c. feta cheese, crumbled

Directions:

1. Using a large pot, bring lightly salted boiling water to a boil. Cook pasta until it is fork-tender.

2. While pasta is cooking, mix tomatoes and beans in a large non-stick skillet. Bring the mixture to a boil over medium high heat.
3. Reduce heat and simmer for about 10 minutes.
4. Add spinach to the skillet and cook for at least two minutes. The spinach should wilt. Stir constantly.
5. Serve sauce over pasta. Sprinkle with feta as desired.

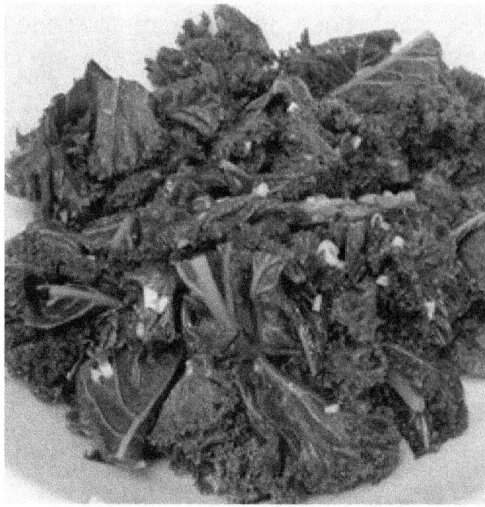

Mediterranean Kale

(ready in about 25 minutes | Serving 6)

Ingredients:

- 12 c. kale, chopped
- 2 tbsp. lemon juice
- 1 tbsp. extra virgin olive oil
- 1 tbsp. garlic, minced
- 1 tsp soy sauce
- Sea salt, to taste
- Freshly ground black pepper, to taste

Directions:

1. Place a steamer insert into a large saucepan. Fill the sauce pan with enough water to come just below the bottom of the steamer.

2. Cover the sauce pan and bring to a boil over high heat.
3. Once boiling, add the kale and cover. Steam until it is just tender. This should take between 7 to 10 minutes.
4. In a large bowl, mix together the remaining ingredients.
5. Toss the steamed kale into the dressing and toss to coat well.

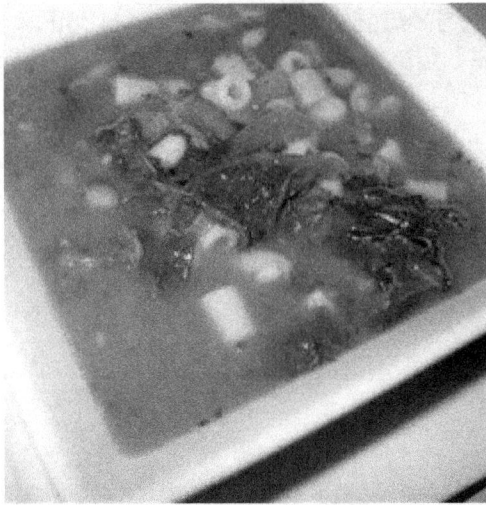

Pasta Fagioli Soup
(ready in about 1 hour 15 minutes | Serving 8)

Ingredients:

- 1 can (28 oz.) diced tomatoes
- 2 cans (14 oz. each) great Northern Beans, undrained
- 1 can (14 oz.) spinach, drained
- 2 cans (14.5 oz. each) chicken broth
- 1 can (8 oz.) tomato sauce
- 3 c. water
- 1 tbsp. garlic, minced
- 8 slices bacon, cooked until crisp and crumbled
- 1 tbsp. dried parsley
- 1 tsp garlic powder
- 1 ½ tsp sea salt
- ½ tsp freshly ground black pepper
- ½ tsp dried basil
- 8 oz. seashell pasta

Directions:

1. In a large stock pot, combine all ingredients except for chees and pasta. Bring mixture to a boil and allow it to simmer for at least 40 minutes
2. Add the pasta and cook uncovered until the pasta is tender. This should take about 10 minutes.
3. Ladle the soup into individual serving bowls. Sprinkle cheese on top.
4. Serve with crusty bread.

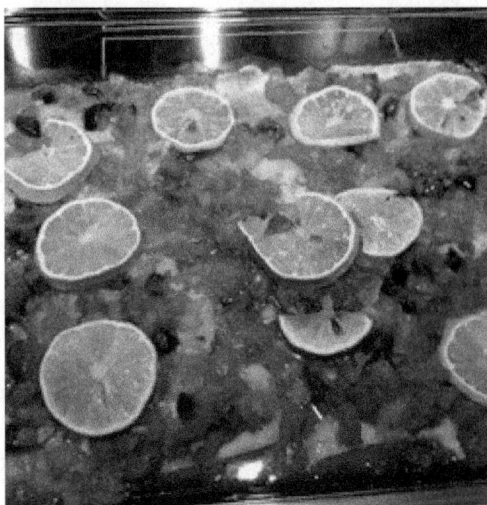

Mediterranean Flounder

(ready in about 45 minutes | Serving 4)

Ingredients:

- 1 lb. flounder fillets
- 5 Roma tomatoes
- ½ Spanish onion, chopped
- ¼ c. white wine of your choice
- ¼ c. capers
- 24 Kalamata olives, pitted and chopped small
- 2 tbsp. extra virgin olive oil
- 2 cloves garlic, peeled and chopped
- 1 pinch Italian seasoning
- 1 tsp. freshly squeezed lemon juice
- 6 leaves fresh basil, chopped
- 6 leaves fresh basil, torn
- 3 tbsp. freshly grated Parmesan cheese

Directions:

1. Preheat oven to 425 degrees F.
2. In a large sauce pan, bring a pot of water to a boil. Stick tomatoes into boiling water and remove them immediately. Place them directly into a medium bowl of ice water. Allow to sit for about 2 minutes and drain. Peel tomatoes and discard the skins. Chop the tomatoes and set aside.
3. In a skillet over medium heat, sauté onion and olive oil together. Cook for about 5 minutes. Stir in tomatoes and Italian seasoning. Allow to cook until the tomatoes are tender. This should take between 5 to 7 minutes.
4. Mix in remaining ingredients, reserving flounder fillets and ½ of the basil.
5. Reduce heat and allow the mixture to cook until the sauce is thickened. This should take about 15 minutes.
6. Place the flounder fillets into a shallow baking dish. Pour the sauce over fish and sprinkle with the remaining basil leaves.
7. Bake the dish for 12 minutes, or until the fish is flaked easily with a fork.

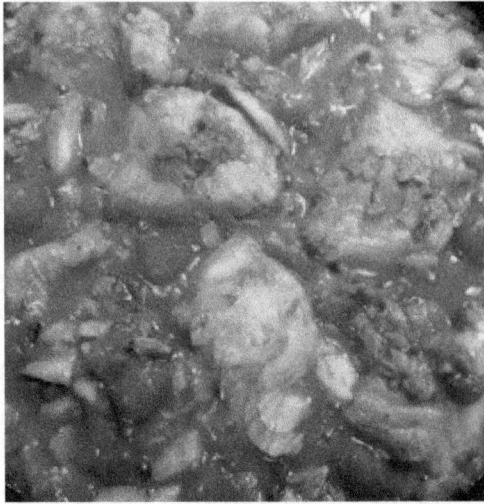

Spanish Cod
(ready in about 35 minutes | Serving 6)

Ingredients:

- 6 cod fillets (4 oz. each)
- ½ c. green olives, chopped
- ¼ c. deli marinated Italian vegetable salad, drained and chopped coarsely
- ¼ c. onion, chopped finely
- 15 cherry or grape tomatoes, halved
- 1 c. tomato sauce of your choice
- 1 tbsp. butter
- 1 tbsp. olive oil
- 2 tbsp. garlic, peeled and chopped
- 1 dash freshly ground black pepper
- 1 dash ground cayenne pepper
- 1 dash smoked paprika

Directions:

1. Heat butter and oil in a large skillet that has been heated over medium high heat.
2. Cook onion and garlic together until they are slightly tender.
3. Add tomato sauce and tomatoes and bring to a simmer.
4. Stir in olives and vegetables. Season the mixture.
5. Cook the fillets in the sauce over medium heat. It should take about 8 minutes for the fillets to reach the right doneness to be flaked with a fork. Serve immediately.

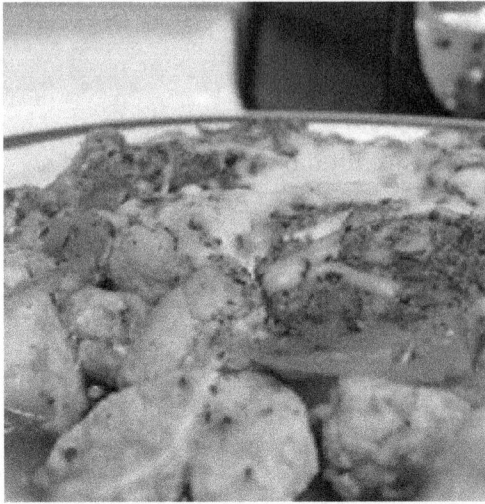

Mediterranean Chicken with Eggplant

(ready in about 1 hour 30 minutes | Serving 4 to 6)

Ingredients:

- 3 eggplants, peeled, cut lengthwise into ½ inch slices
- 6 chicken breast halves, boneless and skinless, diced
- 1 medium onion, diced
- 3 tbsp. olive oil
- 2 tbsp. tomato paste
- ½ c. water
- 2 tsp dried oregano
- Sea salt and pepper, to taste

Directions:

1. Fill a large pot with lightly salted water. Soak eggplant in the water for at least ½ hour.

2. Take eggplant out of the pot and brush with olive oil. Sauté, or grill until it is lightly browned. Place cooked eggplant into a 9 x 13 inch baking dish. Set this dish aside.
3. Sauté chicken and onion over medium heat in a large skillet. Stir in tomato paste and water. Reduce heat and simmer on low for 10 minutes.
4. Meanwhile, preheat oven to 400 degrees F.
5. Pour chicken mixture over the eggplant. Season the dish and cover it with aluminum foil. Bake for 20 minutes.

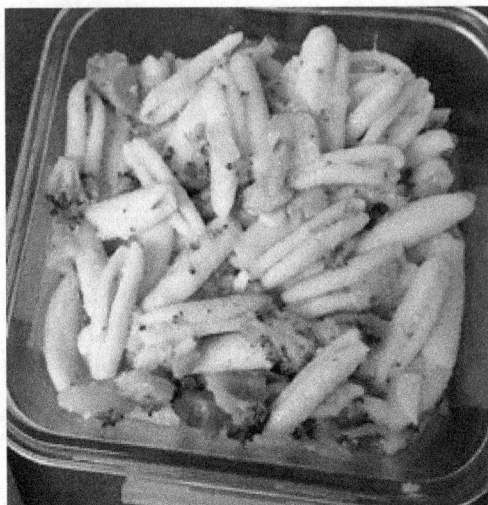

Cavatelli and Broccoli
(ready in about 35 minutes| Serving 12)

Ingredients:

- 3 heads fresh broccoli, cut into small florets
- 1 ½ lb. cavatelli past
- 3 cloves garlic, peeled and minced
- ½ c. olive oil
- 1 tsp. salt
- 1 tsp crushed red pepper flakes
- 2 tbsp. grated Parmesan cheese

Directions:

1. Using a large pot, of lightly salted water, blanch broccoli for 5 minutes. Drain well and set aside.

2. Heat olive oil in a big skillet over medium heat. Cook garlic until it is lightly golden brown. Add broccoli, sauté occasionally for 10 minutes. The broccoli should be tender but slightly crisp when you bite it.
3. Meanwhile, cook pasta in a large pot of lightly salted water. Pasta should be just fork-tender. Drain pasta and place it in a large serving bowl, toss pasta and broccoli together. Season the dish with salt, pepper and pepper flakes.
4. Serve the dish with freshly grated Parmesan cheese.

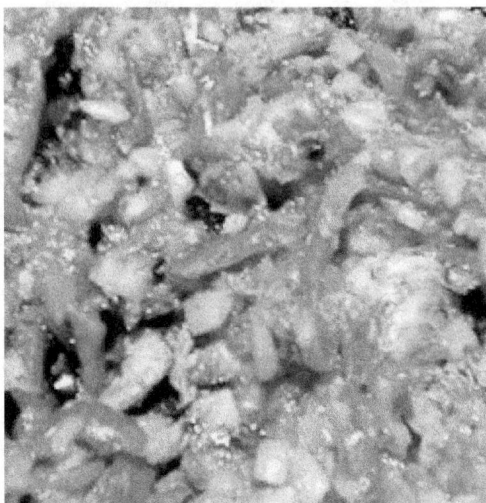

Chicken Costa Brava
(ready in about 40 minutes | Serving 10)

Ingredients:

- 1 can (20 oz.) can pineapple chunks
- 10 chicken breast halves, boneless and skinless
- 1 can (14.5 oz.) stewed tomatoes
- 1 large onion, quartered
- 1 large red bell pepper, sliced thinly
- 2 c. black olives
- ½ c. salsa
- 2 cloves garlic, peeled and minced
- 1 tbsp. vegetable oil
- 1 tsp ground cumin
- 1 tsp ground cinnamon
- 2 tbsp. cornstarch
- 2 tbsp. water
- Salt and pepper to taste

Directions:

1. Drain pineapple and reserve juice. Sprinkle the pineapple with salt.
2. Using a large frying pan, brown the chicken in vegetable oil. Combine cumin and cinnamon. Sprinkle mixture over chicken. Add the onion and garlic and cook until soft. Add the reserved juice, olives, salsa, and tomatoes. Cover the dish and simmer for 25 minutes.
3. Mix the cornstarch with the water, stir into the pan juices. Add in the bell pepper. Allow to simmer until the sauce thickens. Stir in pineapple and continue cooking until it is heated through.

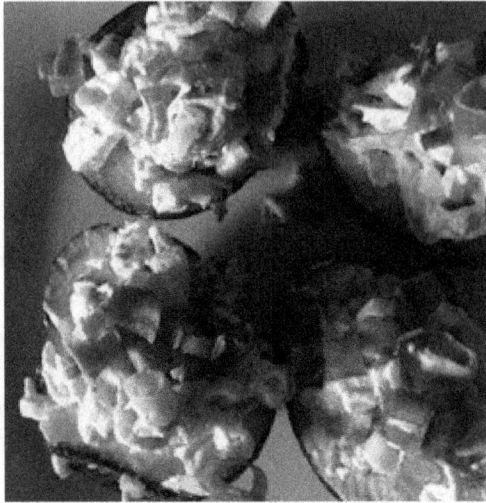

Avocado and Tuna Appetizers
(ready in about 20 minutes | Serving 4)

Ingredients:

- 1 can (12 oz.) solid white tuna that was packed in water, drained
- 2 ripe avocados, halved and pitted
- 4 green onions, minced
- ½ red bell pepper, diced
- 1 dash balsamic vinegar
- Sea salt, to taste
- Freshly ground black pepper, to taste

Directions:

1. Stir together all ingredients, reserving seasoning and enough green onions for garnish. Season to taste.
2. Pack avocado halves with tuna mixture.
3. Garnish with reserved green onion.

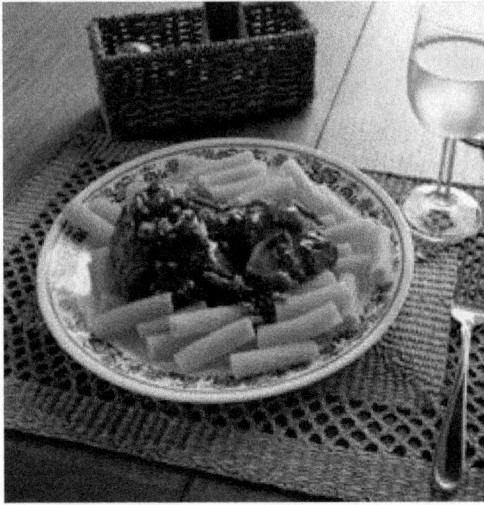

Rosemary and Red Pepper Chicken (slow cooker)
(ready in about 7 hours | Serving 8)

Ingredients:

- 8 skinless, boneless chicken breast halves (4 ounces each)
- 8 oz. turkey sausages, remove casings
- 1 small white onion, sliced into very thin slices
- 1 medium red bell pepper, sliced into very thin slices
- ¼ c. dry vermouth
- 4 large cloves garlic, peeled and minced
- 2 tsp, dried rosemary
- 2 tbsp. cold water
- 1 ½ tbsp. cornstarch
- ½ tsp dried oregano
- ¼ tsp freshly ground black pepper
- ¼ c. fresh parsley, chopped
- Sea salt, to taste

Directions:

1. Using a 5 to 6 quart slow cooker, combine all ingredients, reserving salt and parsley. Mix all ingredients well. Cook on low for 5 to 7 hours, or until chicken is tender and thoroughly cooked.
2. Transfer chicken to a warm, deep platter. Cover to keep warm.
3. Using a small bowl, stir together the cornstarch and water. Increase the temperature to high and cover.
4. Cook until sauce is thickened, stirring 2 to 3 times. This should take about 10 minutes.
5. Season the sauce with salt, to taste. Spoon sauce over chicken sprinkle the top with parsley to garnish.

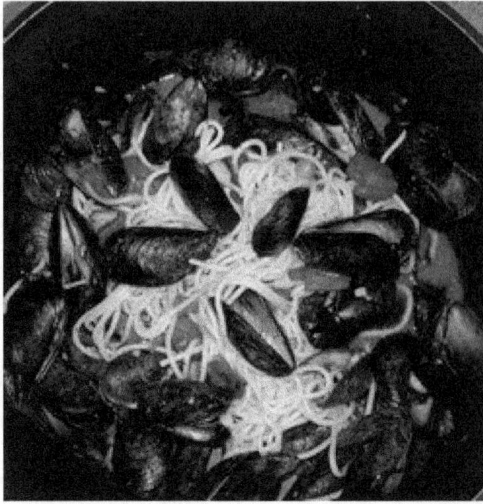

Mussels Marinara di Amore
(ready in about 20 minutes | Serving 4)

Ingredients:

- 1 lb. mussels, cleaned and debeareded
- ½ lb. linguini pasta
- 1 can (14.5 oz.) crushed tomatoes
- ¼ c. white wine of your choice
- 1 tbsp. olive oil
- 1 large clove garlic, minced
- ½ tsp dried oregano
- ½ tsp dried basil
- 1 pinch crushed red pepper flakes
- 1 lemon cut into wedges to use as garnish

Directions:

1. Using a large skillet, heat oil and sauté garlic.
2. Add in tomatoes, red pepper flakes, basil and oregano. Reduce heat to low and allow to simmer for about 5 minutes.
3. Meanwhile, bring a large pot of salted water to a boil. Add the pasta and cook until it is just fork tender. Drain and set aside.
4. Add the mussels and wine to the skillet. Crank the heat up to high for about 5 minutes, or until the shells of the mussels open. Discard any that do not open.
5. Pour sauce over hot pasta. Sprinkle the dish with parsley and squeeze a lemon wedge all over.
6. Serve garnished with remaining lemon.

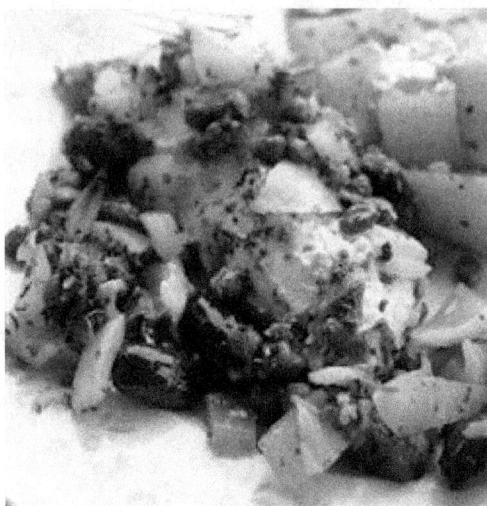

Easy Mediterranean Fish
(ready in about 45 minutes | Serving 4)

Ingredients:

- 4 fillets halibut, 4 ounces each
- 1 tbsp. Greek seasoning
- 1 large tomato, diced
- 1 large onion, diced
- 1 jar (5 oz.) pitted Kalamata olives
- 1/4c. capers
- ¼ c. olive oil
- 1 tbsp. lemon juice
- Sea salt and freshly ground pepper, to taste

Directions:

1. Preheat oven to 350 degrees F.
2. Put halibut fillets on a sheet aluminum foil and season with Greek seasoning.
3. Combine remaining ingredients in a bowl. Spoon mixture over fish.
4. Carefully seal all of the edges of the foil sheet in a way that creates a large packet. Put the package on a baking sheet.
5. Bake for 30 to 40 minutes or until fish is easy to flake with a fork.

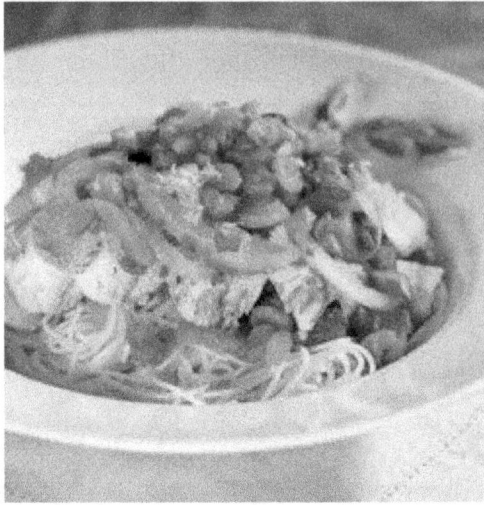

Sicilian Lemon Chicken with Raisin-Tomato Sauce

(ready in about 1 hour 30 minutes | Serving 4)

Ingredients:

- 4 boneless, skinless chicken breasts, 6 ounces each
- ¾ c. golden raisins
- 1 medium white onion, halved and sliced very thin
- 1 can (15 oz.) diced tomatoes, drained well
- 1 lb. angel hair pasta
- ¼ c. shaved Parmesan cheese
- 3 tbsp. extra virgin olive oil
- 2 tbsp. pine nuts
- 2 tbsp. black olives, chopped well
- 2 tbsp. fresh basil, julienned
- 1 tbsp. garlic, minced
- 1 tbsp. extra virgin olive oil
- 1 tbsp. balsamic vinegar
- 2 bay leaves

- 1 tsp white sugar
- ¼ tsp. dried oregano
- ¼ tsp. cayenne pepper
- 4 sprigs fresh basil
- Zest and juice of 1 lemon
- Sea salt and pepper to taste

Directions:

1. Soak raisins in warm water for about 10 minutes, they will plump up. Drain raisins and set aside.
2. Heat 3 tbsp. of oil in a pan over medium high heat. Stir in onion, garlic, pine nuts and olives. Season using bay leaves, oregano and cayenne. Cook mixture until the onions have started to soften and they begin to turn golden in color. This should take about 5 minutes. Stir the tomatoes in and season to taste with salt and pepper.
3. Cook for 5 additional minutes. Toss in raisins, vinegar and sugar. Stir occasionally to prevent burning until the sauce thickens. This should take about 5 more minutes.
4. Remove bay leaves and stir in basil. Cover and keep warm.
5. Bring a large pot of water to a boil. Salt the water lightly. Add pasta and cook for between 8 to 10 minutes, or until it is fork tender. Drain well.
6. While the pasta is cooking, heat the 1 tbsp. olive oil in a skillet over medium heat. While you are waiting for the oil to heat up, toss the chicken in lemon juice. Cook chicken in oil until it is tender, golden brown and the juices run clear. This should take about 15 minutes on each side.
7. Transfer the chicken to a warm plate and let it rest for at least 5 minutes.
8. Before serving, slice each piece of chicken against the grain. Divide pasta into four bowls that are wide and shallow.

9. Fan chicken over pasta and spoon sauce over top. Sprinkle with zest, cheese and basil to garnish.

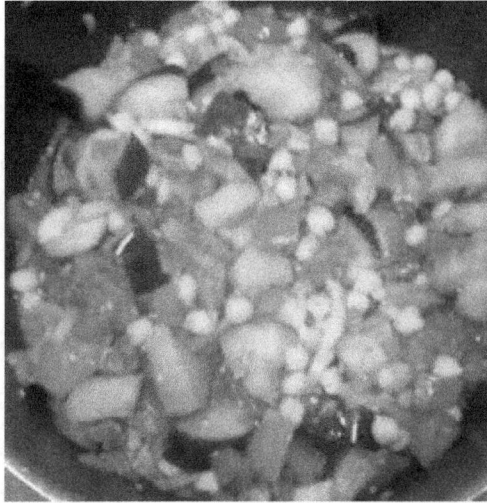

Mediterranean Vegetable Stew
(ready in about 35 minutes | Serving 6)

Ingredients:

- 1 small eggplant, cut into 1 inch chunks
- 1 c. chopped red onion
- 2 c. chopped green pepper
- 1 can (15 oz.) chickpeas, drained and rinsed
- 1 can (28 oz.) crushed tomatoes
- ½ c. Kalamata olives
- 1 can (28 oz.) crushed tomatoes
- 1 tbsp. olive oil, divided
- 1 c. sliced mushrooms
- 2 large cloves garlic, peeled and crushed
- 1 c. coarsely chopped parsley
- 1 tbsp. fresh rosemary, chopped

Directions:

1. Using a large skillet, heat 1 tbsp. of the oil. Sauté onion and pepper until they are soft. This should take about 10 minutes
2. Add 1 tbsp. of oil. Add garlic, mushrooms and eggplant. Simmer, stirring occasionally until the eggplant becomes soft. Be careful not to overcook it because you do not want the eggplant to become mushy.
3. Add in remaining ingredients, reserving parsley and feta cheese. Simmer the mixture for about 10 minutes. Stir in parsley and sprinkle feta cheese over the stew if you desire.

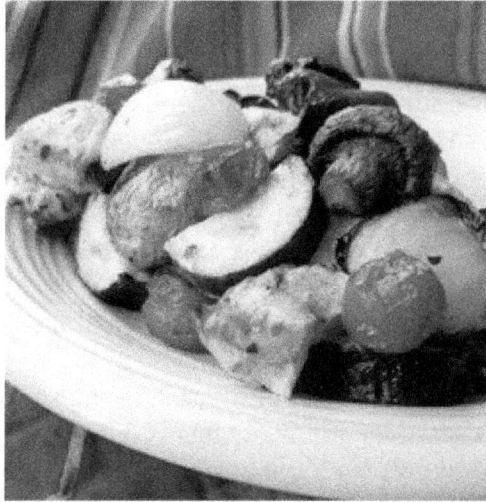

Greek Island Chicken Shish Kabobs
(ready in about 2 hours 30 minutes | Serving 6 skewers)

Ingredients:

- 2 lbs. chicken breasts, skinless and boneless, cut into 1 ½ inch pieces
- 12 cherry tomatoes
- 12 fresh mushrooms
- 1 large onion, quartered and separated into slices
- 2 large bell peppers, cut into 1 inch pieces
- 2 cloves garlic, peeled and minced
- ¼ c. lemon juice
- ¼ c. olive oil
- ¼ c. white vinegar
- 1 tsp ground cumin
- 1 tsp dried oregano
- ½ tsp dried thyme
- ¼ tsp salt

- 6 wooden skewers

Directions:

1. Using a ceramic bowl, whisk together olive oil, lemon juice, vinegar, garlic, cumin, oregano, thyme, salt and pepper. Add chicken and toss to coat evenly and allow to marinate in the refrigerator for between 2 hours and overnight.
2. Soak wooden skewers in water for at least 30 minutes, right before you plan to use them.
3. Preheat a grill for medium-high heat. Oil the grate lightly to prevent sticking.
4. Take the chicken out of the marinade and shake off excess liquid. Discard the marinade that is left over.
5. Tread the skewers, alternating between chicken, bell pepper, onion, cherry tomatoes and mushrooms.
6. Cook skewers on the grill, turning frequently until it has been browned on all sides. This should take about 10 minutes

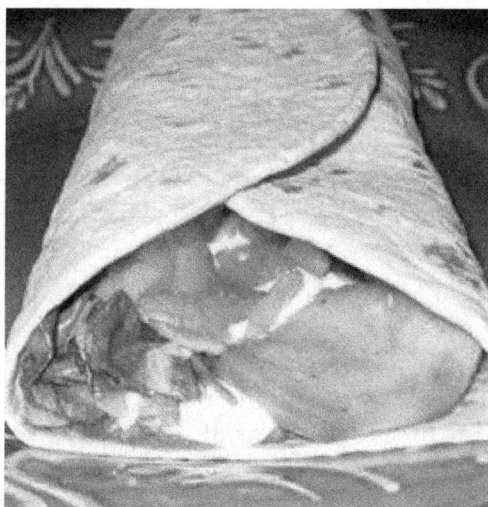

Mediterranean Wrap

(ready in about 35 minutes | Serving 4)

Ingredients:

- 1 eggplant, thinly sliced
- 1 red onion, thinly sliced
- 1 zucchini, thinly sliced
- 1 red bell pepper, sliced
- 4 whole grain tortillas
- 1 large avocado, sliced
- ¼ lb. fresh mushrooms
- ¼ c. goat cheese
- ¼ c. basil pesto
- 1 tbsp. olive oil
- Sea salt and ground black pepper, to taste

Directions:

1. Place all vegetables in a large container that has a tight fitting lid. Drizzle olive oil over vegetables and season with sea salt and ground black pepper. Place the lid on and shake vigorously until all vegetables are well coated.
2. Heat a grill pan or skillet on medium high heat. Place seasoned vegetables in preheated pan. Stir the vegetables, being careful not to burn them, for about 10 minutes.
3. Spread each tortilla with 1 tbsp. goat cheese and 1 tbsp. pesto.
4. Divide the sliced avocado between the tortillas and top with vegetables. Fold the bottom of each tortilla toward the center, followed by rolling each tortilla into a tight wrap.

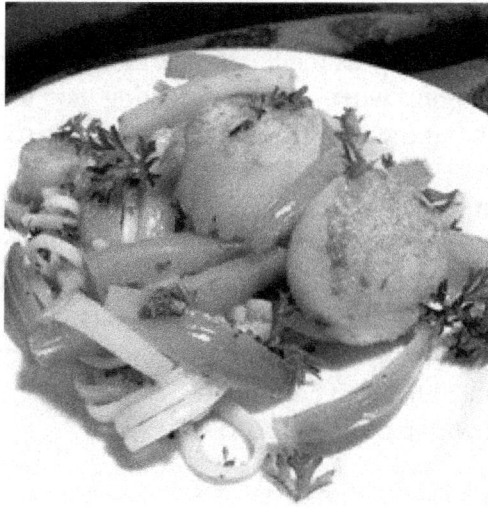

Pan Seared Scallops with Peppers and Onions
(ready in about 45 minutes | Serving 4)

Ingredients:

- 1 lb. large scallops
- 1 red onion, chopped coarsely
- 1 large bell pepper, chopped coarsely
- 1 can (2 ounce) anchovy fillets, minced
- 1/3 c. extra virgin olive oil
- 2 cloves garlic, sliced thinly
- 1 tsp lime zest, minced
- 1 ½ tsp lemon zest, minced
- 1 pinch sea salt
- 8 sprigs fresh parsley

Directions:

1. Heat olive oil and minced anchovies in a skillet over medium high heat. Stir oil as the anchovies dissolve. Once anchovies are at the point where they are sizzling, add the scallops and cook leaving the scallops still for 2 minutes so that they can sear.
2. Meanwhile, toss in remaining ingredients in a bowl. Once scallops are ready, sprinkle the vegetable mixture onto the searing scallops. Continue to cook until the scallops are cooked on both sides, for 2 minutes longer.
3. Continue cooking until scallops are browned on both sides, which may take 4 to 5 minutes.
4. Garnish with parsley and serve.

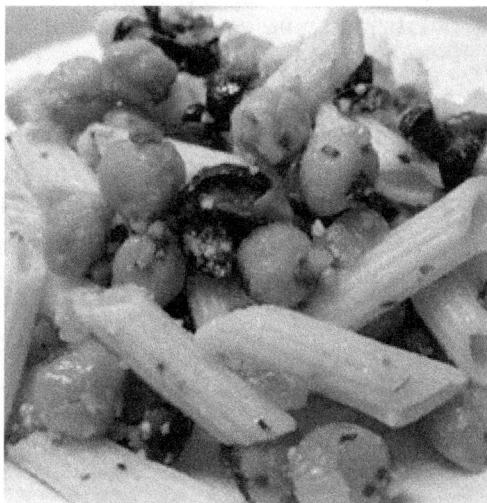

Pasta Chickpea Salad

(Total Time 2 hours| Servings 6)

Ingredients:

- 1 lb. rotelle pasta
- 2 tbsp. extra virgin olive oil
- ½ c. cured olives, chopped
- 2 tbsp. oregano, minced
- 2 tbsp. fresh parsley, chopped
- 1 can (15 oz.) garbanzo beans
- ¼ c. red wine vinegar
- ½ c. parmesan cheese, grated
- Sea salt and freshly ground pepper, to taste

Directions:

1. In a large pot, bring some lightly salted water to a boil. Add pasta and cook until fork tender. Drain completely, rinse, and place in the refrigerator to chill.
2. Using a large skillet, heat olive oil over medium low heat. Add olives, chickpeas, oregano, parsley, and scallions. Cook over low for about 20 minutes. Set aside and allow to cool.
3. Using a large bowl, toss pasta with bean mixture. Add remaining ingredients, reserving salt, pepper and olive oil for serving.
4. Allow to sit in the refrigerator overnight so that the flavors have a chance to meld.

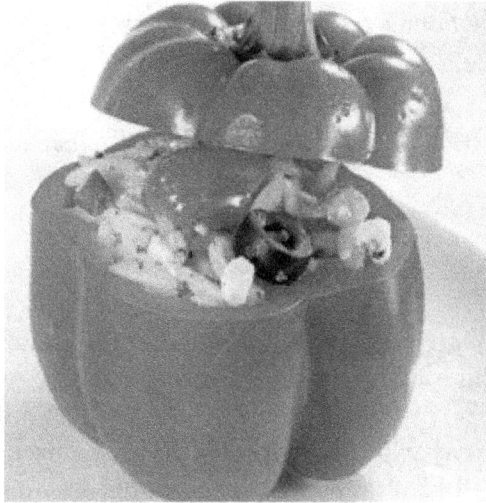

Mediterranean Chicken and Orzo Salad in Red Pepper Cups

(Total Time 1 hour 15 minutes| Servings 4)

Ingredients:

- ¼ Cup – Olive oil
- ½ lbs. – Orzo pasta uncooked
- 1 tsp. – Dijon mustard
- 1/3 Cup – Red wine vinegar
- ¾ tsp. – Oregano, dried
- ¾ tsp. – Garlic powder
- ¾ tsp. – Onion Powder
- ¾ tsp. – Basil, dried
- ¼ tsp. – Black pepper, ground
- ½ tsp. – Salt
- ¼ Cup – Black olives, cut in half lengthwise
- ½ Cup – Grape tomatoes, cut in half

- 1 – Grilled chicken breast half, diced
- 2 oz. – Feta cheese crumbled
- 4 Sprigs – Fresh oregano
- 2 – Red bell peppers, cut in half lengthwise and seeded

Directions:

1. Bring a large pot full of water and lightly salted to a rolling boil on high heat. Stir in your orzo when the water starts boiling and bring the water back to a boil. Stir the orzo occasionally while uncovered until you have cooked pasta that is still firm to the bite. This should take around 11 minutes. Pour your water and pasta into a colander and let sit in the sink. When well drained pour the pasta into a bowl and place in the refrigerator to cool.
2. Whisk the red wine vinegar, olive oil, Dijon mustard, oregano, garlic powder, basil, salt, onion powder and pepper together in a small bowl. Mix your now cooked orzo, olives, tomatoes, chicken breast, and feta cheese in a large bowl. Pour your Dijon dressing mix over the orzo mixture and mix them together so that it is coated evenly. Spoon the mixture into the halves of red peppers and garnish with your sprig of oregano.

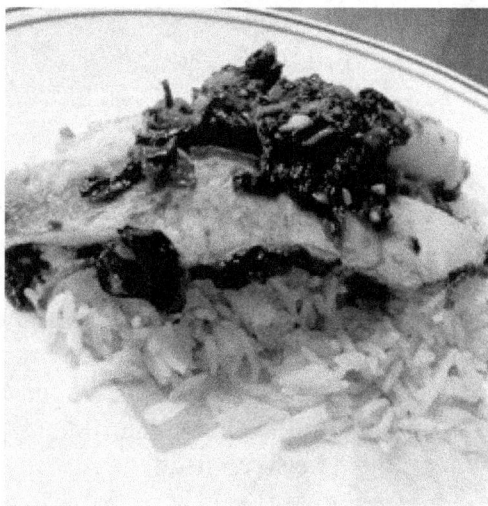

Tilapia Feta Florentine

(Total Time is about 55 minutes | Servings 4)

Ingredients:

- ¼ Cup – Onion, chopped
- 2 tsps. – Olive oil
- 2 Bags (9 oz.) – Spinach, fresh
- 1 Clove – Garlic, minced
- 2 tbsps. – Feta cheese, crumbled
- ¼ Cup – Kalamata olives, sliced
- ½ tsp. – Salt
- ½ tsp. – Lemon rind, grated
- 1/8 tsp. – White pepper
- ¼ tsp. – Oregano, dried
- 2 tbsps. – Butter, melted
- 1 lb. – Tilapia fillets
- 1 Pinch – Paprika

- 2 tsps. – Lemon juice

Directions:

1. Set your oven to preheat at 400 °F
2. Pour your olive oil in a large skillet that has been set on medium heat. Cook your garlic, and onions in the skillet while stirring until the onion has become soft. Add your spinach to the hot skillet, cook and stir until the spinach has become wilted. Stir in your feta cheese, olives, salt, lemon rind, white pepper, and oregano into the spinach mixture. Cook the mixture until the cheese has melted and the mixture is evenly distributed between itself.
3. Take your spinach mixture and spread it into a baking dish that is a 9x13-inch. Lay the tilapia fillets over the top of the spinach mixture. In a small bowl mix your lemon juice and butter and drizzle it over your tilapia. Sprinkle the top with paprika.
4. Place the dish in the preheated oven and bake for 20 to 25 minutes. The tilapia will be opaque in color.

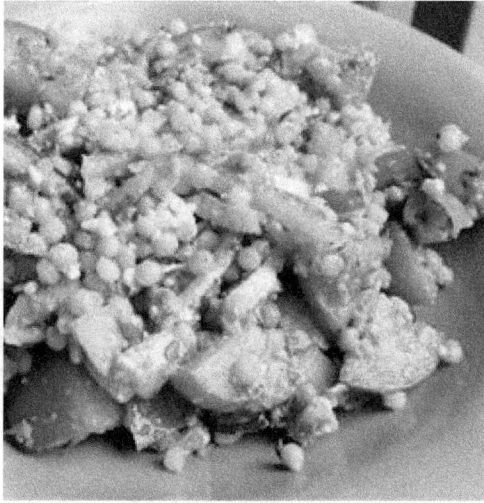

Heirloom Tomato Salad with Pearl Couscous

- (Total Time 1 hour and 30 minutes| Servings 10)

Ingredients:

- 1 tbsp. – Extra-virgin olive oil
- 2 Cups – Vegetable stock
- ½ Cup – Fresh basil leaves, packed
- 1 Cup – Pearl (Israeli) couscous
- 1 Clove – Garlic, crushed
- ¼ Cup – Flat-leaf parsley leaves
- 1 tbsp. – Fresh thyme, chopped
- 1 tbsp. – Fresh oregano
- 4 – Heirloom tomatoes, quartered
- ½ Cup – Green olives, pitted
- 1 – English cucumber, cubed
- 15 – Cherry tomatoes, quartered
- 1 Cup – Feta cheese, crumbled

- ½ Small – Red Onion, thinly sliced
- ½ Cup – Extra-virgin olive oil
- ¼ Cup – White balsamic vinegar
- 1 – Lemon, juiced

Directions:

1. Pour the vegetable stock into a saucepan and simmer on medium heat. Place 1 tbsp. olive oil in a skillet set to medium heat. Mix in the couscous, cooking while stirring until it turns a golden brown. This should take about 10 minutes. Pour the cooked couscous into the hot vegetable stock until the couscous absorbs the stock. This will take about 15 minutes. Scrape out the couscous into a mixing bowl and use a fork to fluff. Set the couscous to the side to cool off.
2. Use a food processor and place the parsley, basil, garlic, thyme, oregano, and olive into it. Pulse the herbs until they become chopped coarsely. Pour the herbs into the couscous along with the cherry tomatoes, heirloom tomatoes, red onion, cucumber, ad feta cheese. Drizzle the ½ cup olive oil, vinegar, and lemon juice over the top and stir until mixed evenly.

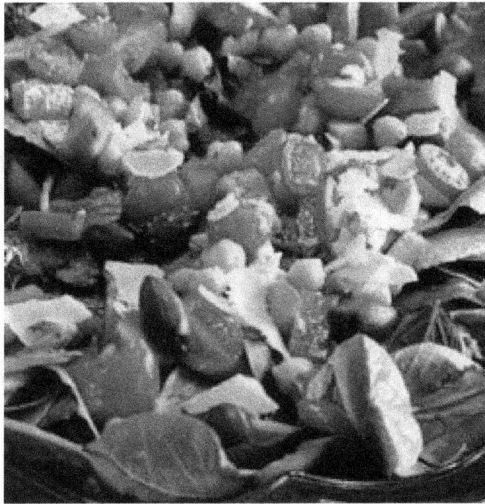

Italian Panzanella Bread Salad
(Total Time 1 hour 45 minutes | Servings10)

Ingredients:

- 3 tbsps. – Garlic flavored olive oil
- 8 oz. – Country style white bread, cut into 1 inch cubes
- 1 Can (15 oz.) – Garbanzo beans, rinsed and drained
- 1/3 Cup – Green bell peppers, chopped
- 2 Cups – Red or yellow teardrop tomatoes, halved
- 1 Small – Red onion, cut into ¾ inch slices
- 1/3 Cup – Red bell pepper, chopped
- 1/3 Cup – Basil pesto
- 10 – Kalamata olives, pitted and halved
- 1 tbsp. – Fresh rosemary, minced
- ¼ Cup – Balsamic vinegar
- 4 oz. – Goat cheese, crumbled

- ¼ tsp. – Black pepper
- ¼ Cup – Pine nuts, poasted
- 1 Head – Green or red leaf lettuce

Directions:

1. Preheat your oven to 350 °F.
2. Toss your bread cubes in the olive oil, coating them evenly. Sprinkle it with salt and toss to mix. Spread the bread cubes out over a baking sheet and place in the oven to bake until it becomes a golden brown. This will take about 12 minutes. Remove the sheet from the oven and allow the bread to cool.
3. Mix the tomatoes, garbanzo beans, Kalamata olives, and onions in a large bowl. Whisk the balsamic vinegar, pesto, pepper and rosemary in a separate bowl. Now toss the tomatoes mixture with the pesto mixture and let marinade at room temperature for about 1 hour.
4. Toss the goat cheese and bread cubes in with the tomato mixture coating them evenly. Place a couple lettuce leave on a serving platter and shred any remaining lettuce to make a pile in the middle of the serving dish. Spread the mixture of bread on top of the lettuce and top with the toasted pine nuts.

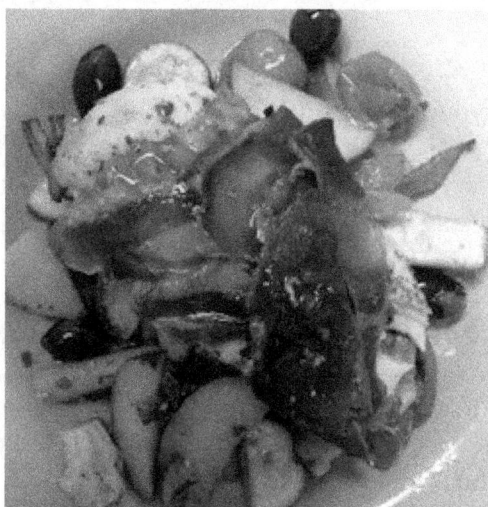

Parma Wrapped Chicken with Mediterranean Vegetables

(Total Time 1 hour 25 minutes| Servings 2)

Ingredients:

- 1 – Zucchini, halved lengthwise and cut into 1 inch slices
- ½ lb. – Baby red potatoes, cut in half
- 2 – Red bell peppers, cut into 1 inch pieces
- 1 – Red onion, cut into 1/2-inch thick wedge
- 2 tbsps. Garlic, minced
- 12 – Cherry tomatoes
- ¼ tsp. – Red pepper flakes, crushed
- ½ tsp. – Thyme leaves, dried
- 2 tbsps. – Olive oil
- Salt and freshly ground pepper to taste
- 4 (1/2 oz.) – Prosciutto di parma, sliced thinly

- 2 (5 oz.) Boneless chicken breast halves, skinless

Directions:

1. Preheat your oven at 400 °F
2. Mix zucchini, potatoes, bell peppers, onion, and tomatoes in a large bowl; add thyme, garlic, and red pepper flakes. Toss the vegetable mixture and season with pepper and salt. Coat the top of the vegetables with olive oil and toss them to evenly coat them. Pour this mixture into a glass baking dish and place in the preheated oven. Bake in the oven for about 15 minutes.
3. Season the chicken with pepper and salt. Wrap two slices of prosciutto around each chicken breast and use a toothpick to keep them in place. Place the wrapped chicken on top of the vegetables and continue to bake until the chicken is fully cooked. This will take about 30 minutes.
4. Split the meal in half and arrange them on two plates with the chicken sliced into 5 slices and placing the chicken on top of the vegetables.

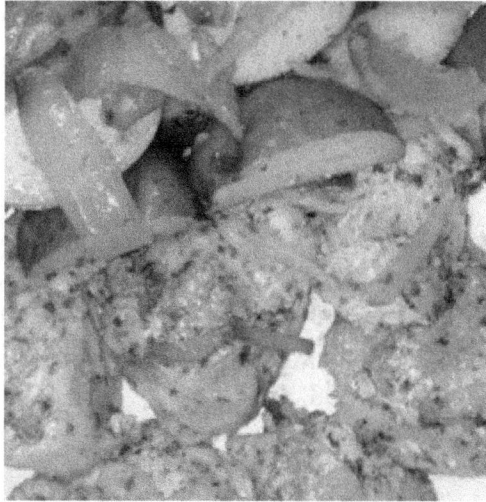

Lemony Mediterranean Chicken

(Total Time 1 hour and 30 minutes| Servings4)

Ingredients:

- 2 tbsps. – Fresh lemon juice
- ¼ Cup – Olive oil
- 4 Large Cloves – Garlic, pressed
- 2 tbsps. – Fresh lemon zest
- ¾ tsp. – Salt
- 4 – Boneless chicken breast halves, skinless
- ½ tsp. – Coarsely ground black pepper
- 1 – Red bell pepper, cut into 1 – inch wide strips
- 9 – Baby red potatoes, halved
- 1 – Lemon, thinly sliced
- 1 – Red onion, cut into 1 – inch wedges

Directions:

1. Preheat your oven at 400 °F
2. Mix lemon juice, olive oil, garlic, lemon zest, salt, oregano and black pepper in a bowl. Fill a 9x13-inch baking dish with your chicken breast. Use a basting brush and brush the mixture of lemon juice over the chicken.
3. In a bowl place your red bell pepper strips, potatoes, lemon slices, and red onion and pour the rest of the mixture of lemon juice on top of the vegetables. Toss the vegetables and lemon mixture together to coat evenly. Move the vegetable and lemon slices are around the edges of the baking dish and chicken is in the middle..
4. Allow to bake in the oven for 30 minutes and brush the vegetables and chicken with pan drippings. Now bake until chicken has browned and it no longer has red juices or reads 160 °F at the chicken's thickest part.

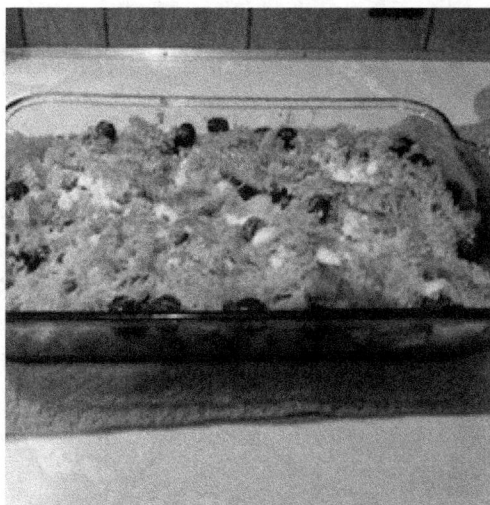

Greek God Pasta

(Total Time 50 minutes| Servings 6)

Ingredients:

- 1 Can (16 oz.) – Tomatoes, peeled, diced and drained
- 1 Pack (16 oz.) Whole wheat rotini pasta
- ¼ Cup – Green onion, chopped
- 2 tbsps. – Green bell pepper, chopped
- 1 tsp. – Basil, dried
- 3 Cups – Tomato sauce
- 1 Cup – Black olives, sliced
- 1 tsp. – Oregano, dried
- 2 tbsps. – Feta cheese, crumbled
- ½ Cup – Mozzarella cheese, shredded
- 2 tbsps. – Feta cheese, crumbled

Directions:

1. Preheat your oven at 400 °F
2. Fill a large pot with lightly salted water and bring to a boil. Add the rotini pasta, cooking it until it is al dente. This should take about 8 minutes. Drain the pasta and place it in a deep casserole dish.
3. Stir green pepper, tomatoes, olives, green onion and tomato sauce in with the pasta. Season the pasta with oregano and basil and mix well until blended evenly. Sprinkle the feta and mozzarella cheese over the top.
4. Place the casserole dish in the preheated oven and bake for 30 minutes. When cheese is melted and bubbly remove the dish and allow to set for 10 minutes to allow for cooling time.

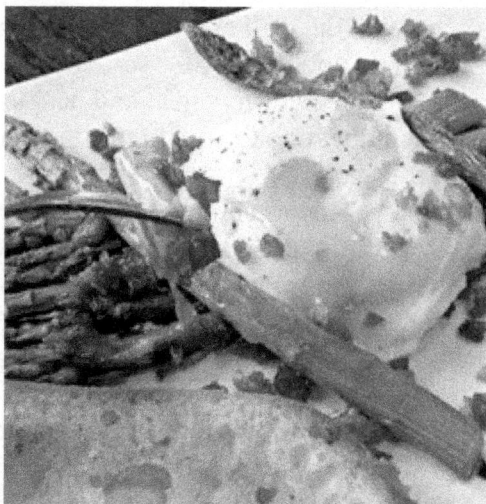

Roasted Asparagus Prosciutto and Egg
(Total Time 40 minutes | Servings4)

Ingredients:

- 1 tbsp. – Extra-virgin olive oil
- 1 Bunch – Fresh asparagus trimmed
- 2 oz. – prosciutto, minced
- 1 tbsp. – olive oil
- 1 tsp. – Distilled white vinegar
- Ground black pepper
- 4 eggs
- 1 Pinch of salt
- 1 Pinch – Ground black pepper
- ½ - Lemon, zested and juiced

Directions:

1. Preheat your oven to about 425 °F. Lay asparagus down in the bottom of a baking dish and use 1 tbsp. extra-virgin olive oil to drizzle over top.
2. Place a skillet on medium-low heat and heat up 1 tbsp. olive oil. Add, prosciutto; stir and cook until it is rendered and golden. This will take about 3 to 4 minutes. Drizzle the oil and prosciutto over the asparagus. Season the asparagus with black pepper and mix them by tossing them. Roast the asparagus in the oven for about 10 minutes. Toss the Asparagus again and return them to the oven. Remove them when they become tender and firm. This will take about 5 minutes.
3. Fill a large saucepan with water up to 2 to 3 inches and bring to a boil. Lower the heat so that it is on medium-low, throw in a pinch of salt and pour in vinegar. Crack open both egg without breaking the yolk and slide it in the water. Poach the eggs until the it is cooked almost to the point the yolks are become thick but are not solid. This will take about 4 to 6 minutes. Remove the egg and gently blot it dry. Transfer the poached eggs to a warm plate.
4. Drizzle lemon juice over the asparagus and transfer the asparagus to the plates. Lay the poached egg over the top and add a pinch of your lemon zest. Season it all with some black pepper.

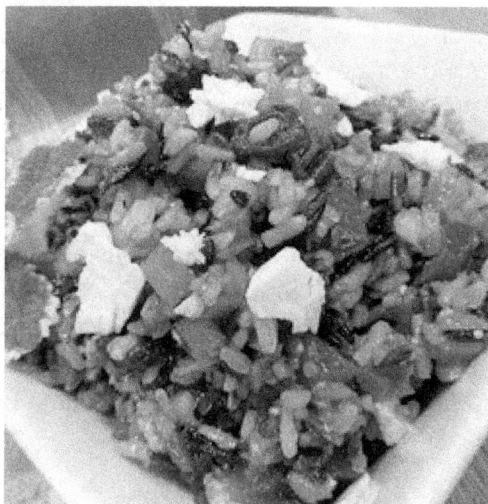

Mediterranean Brown Rice Salad

(Total Time 1 hour| Servings 6)

Ingredients:

- 3 Cups – Water
- 1 ½ Cups – Uncooked brown rice
- 1 Cup – Frozen green peas, thawed
- 1 – Red bell pepper, thinly sliced
- ¼ - Sweet onion, chopped
- ½ Cup – Raisins
- ½ Cup – Kalamata olives, chopped
- ¼ Cup – Balsamic vinegar
- ½ Cup – Vegetable oil
- Salt and Ground black pepper to taste
- 1 ¼ Tsps. – Dijon mustard
- ¼ Cup – Feta cheese

Directions:

1. Bring water and brown rice to a boil over high heat in a saucepan. Lower the heat to medium-low and simmer covered until the rice becomes tender and liquid has been absorbed. This should take about 45 to 50 minutes.
2. In a separate bowl mix the peas, red bell pepper, onion, raisins, and olives together.
3. Whisk vinegar, vegetable oils, and mustard in a separate bowl to create the balsamic dressing.
4. Stir the balsamic dressing and brown rice into the vegetable mixture and season with black pepper and salt.
5. Use the feta cheese to top the vegetables and rice.

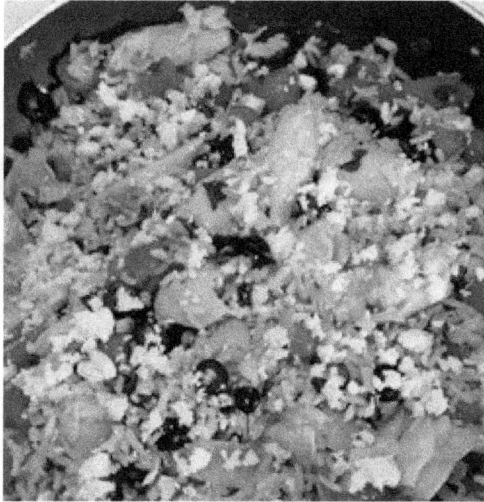

Mediterranean Fried Rice
(Total Time 25 minutes | Servings 4)

Ingredients:

- 1 Clove – Garlic, minced
- 2 Tbsps. – Olive oil
- 1 Pack (10 oz.) – Frozen chopped spinach, thawed and drained
- 1 ½ Cups – Cooked rice
- 1 jar (4 oz.) – Roasted red peppers, drained and chopped
- 1 jar (6 oz.) – Marinated artichoke hearts drained and quartered
- ½ Cup – Geta cheese, crumbled with herbs.

Directions:

1. Place a skillet on medium heat and heat up oil. Stir garlic into the hot oil and cook until brown. This will take about 2 minutes. Stir your rice in and cook until grains of rice are separate and hot. Stir repeatedly for 2 more minutes. Add in your spinach and cook thoroughly for 3 minutes.
2. Stir your roasted red peppers and artichoke hearts into the mixture and cook for 2 minutes. Remove from heat and mix in the feta cheese.

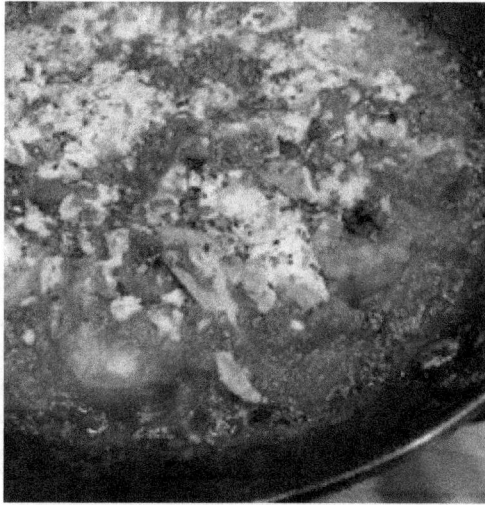

Shrimps Saganaki
(Total Time 40 minutes| Servings 4)

Ingredients:

- 1 – Onion, chopped
- 1 lb. – Medium shrimp, with shells
- 1 Cup – White wine
- 2 Tbsps. – Fresh Parsley, chopped
- ¼ Tsp. – Garlic powder
- 1 Can (14.5 oz.) – Diced tomatoes, drained
- 1 Pack (8 oz.) Feta cheese, cubed
- ¼ Cup – Olive oil
- Salt and pepper to taste

Directions:
1. In a large saucepan bring 2 inches of water to a boil. Add in the shrimp and make sure the water just covers them. Boil the

shrimp for 5 minutes and drain. Set the drained liquid to the side.

2. In a saucepan heat about 2 tbsps. Add in your onions and cook while stirring until soft. Mix in the wine, parsley, garlic powder, tomatoes, and olive oil that is left. Simmer the mixture for 30 minutes while stirring continuously. The sauce should become thickened.

3. While you are simmering your sauce, remove the legs and shell from the shrimp and leave the tail and head on.

4. Once the sauce has thickened stir the shrimp liquid and shrimp into it. Bring the mixture to a simmer, cooking for 5 minutes. Remove from the heat and add in your feta cheese. Let the mixture stand while the feta cheese melts and serve while warm.

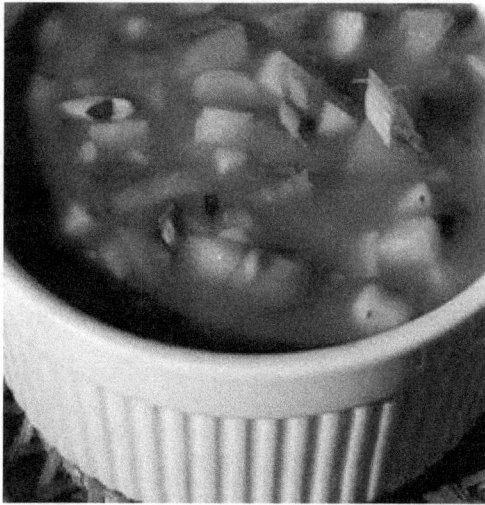

Fresh Market Gazpacho
(Total Time 10 | Servings 2 1/2)

Ingredients:

- 1 can (15.5 oz.) – Garbanzo beans, drained and rinsed
- 5 Large – Roma tomatoes, diced
- 1 – Cucumber, peeled, seeded, and diced
- 1 Stalk – Celery, diced
- 2 Tbsps. – Sweet onion, finely chopped
- 2 – Green onion, chopped
- ½ - Red bell pepper, diced
- ¼ Cup – Fresh parsley, chopped
- ½ - Yellow bell pepper, diced
- 1 can (46 Fluid oz.) – Tomato juice
- 1 Clove – Garlic, minced
- 1 Pinch – Tarragon, dried
- 1 tsp. – Curry powder

- 1 Dash – Hot pepper sauce
- Freshly ground black pepper to taste

Directions:- Lemon, juiced

1. Mix garbanzo beans, tomatoes, cucumber, celery, sweet onion, green onions, yellow bell pepper, red bell pepper, garlic, and lemon juice in a large glass bowl. Pour the tomato juice in and Season with tarragon, curry powder, and hot pepper sauce, Place in the refrigerator to chill for 2 hours.

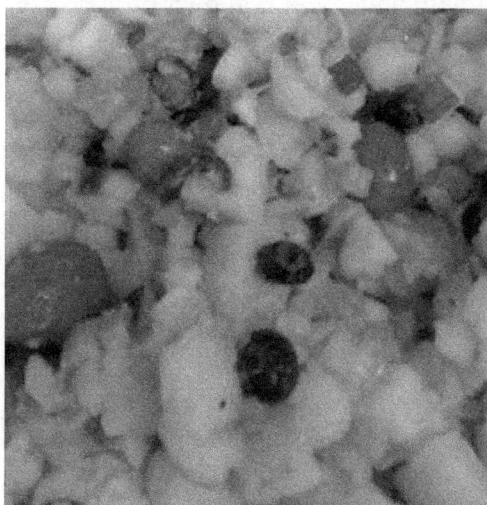

Mom's Italian Potato Salad
(Total Time 1 hour and 45 minutes | Servings 6)

Ingredients:

- 1 Large – Cucumber, chopped
- 5 Large – Yukon gold potatoes
- 1 Large – Red Onion, chopped
- 5 Stalks – Celery, chopped
- ¼ Cup – Olive oil
- ¾ Cup – Green olives with pimento, chopped
- ¼ Tsp. – Garlic powder
- ½ Cup – Red wine vinegar
- Salt and ground black pepper to taste

Directions:

1. Use a large saucepan and place the potatoes into it while covering with water and boil over high heat. Simmer the potatoes on medium for 15 and become tender. Use a colander and drain the potatoes. Cut the potatoes into 1-inch cubes.
2. In a large bowl combine the cucumber, potatoes, onion, celery, and olives.
3. Whisk the red wine vinegar, olive oil, and garlic powder in to a small bowl. Mix the dressing over the vegetables and potatoes. Season with pepper and salt. Place in the refrigerator to chill before you serve.

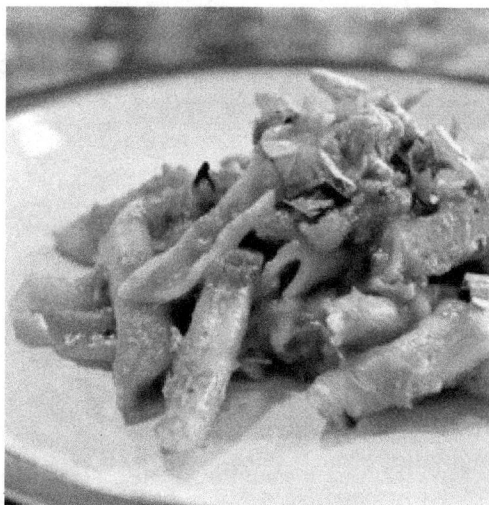

Ziti With Olives and Sun-Dried Tomatoes

(Total Time | Servings 6)

Ingredients:

- 1/3 Cup – Sun-dried tomatoes, chopped
- 1 Pack (16 oz.) – Ziti pasta
- ¼ Cup – Parsley, chopped
- 1/3 Cup – Black Greek olives, pitted and sliced
- 2 – Anchovy fillets, diced
- 2 Tbsps. – Olive oil
- 2 Tsps. – Minced garlic

Directions:

1. Boil your pasta in a large pot of salted water so that the noodle is al dente.
2. Place the sun-dried tomatoes, olive oil, olives, garlic and anchovy fillets in a large bowl.

3. Drain the water from the pasta and pour the pasta into the large bowl with the tomato mix and toss before serving.

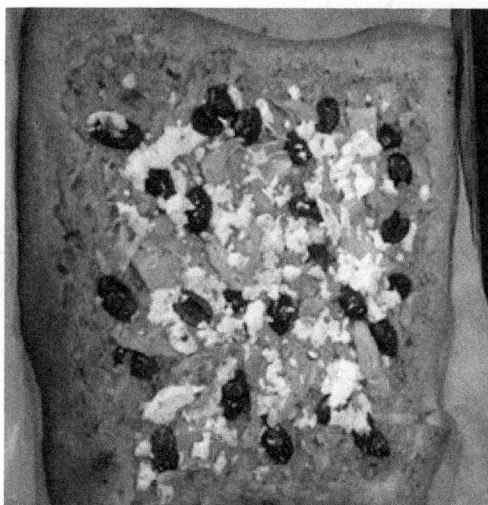

Mediterranean Whole Wheat Pizza
(Total Time 25 minutes| Servings 1 pizza)

Ingredients:

- 1 jar (4 oz.) – Basil pesto
- 1 – Whole wheat pizza crust
- 2 Tbsps. – Kalamata olives, chopped
- ½ Cup – Artichoke hearts, drained and pulled apart
- ¼ Cup – Feta cheese, crumbled
- 2 Tbsps. – Pepperoncini, sliced and drained

Directions:
1. Preheat your oven at 450 °F
2. Flour a flat area to place your pizza crust on and spread pesto over the top. Place pieces of the artichoke hearts on top of the pesto; scatter pepperoncini slices and Kalamata on top of the pizza. Sprinkle crumbled feta cheese over the top.

3. Place the pizza in the oven to bake so that the crust becomes crispy and you have melted feta cheese. This will take about 10 to 12 minutes.

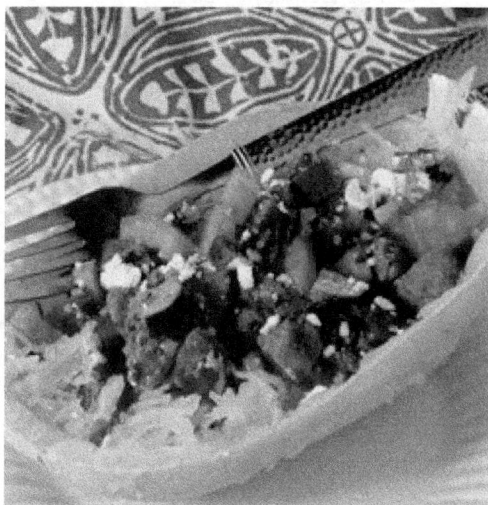

Spaghetti Squash Mediterranean-Style
(Total Time 1 hour and 45 minutes | Servings 4)

Ingredients:

- 1 – Spaghetti squash, halved lengthwise and seeded
- Cooking spray
- 3 (4 oz.) Italian sausage links, castings removed
- 2 Tbsps. – Olive oil, divided
- 3 Cloves – Garlic, minced
- 2 – Spring onions, finely chopped
- 1 – Red bell pepper, seeded and diced
- 1 – Zucchini, diced
- 4 oz. – Feta cheese, crumbled or more to taste
- 1 Tbsp. – Italian seasoning
- 1 Pinch – Lemon pepper, or to taste
- Sea salt to taste
- 1 Tbsp. – Fresh parsley, chopped

- 1 Small – tomato, finely chopped

Directions:

1. Preheat your oven at 350 °F. Use cooking spray to coat a large baking dish.
2. Place your squash in the baking dish cut side down.
3. Place the baking dish in the oven to bake for 45 minutes or until the squash has become tender. Flip the squash to the other side and bake for an additional 5 minutes. Remove the squash and scrape the dish free of the strands and place them in a large bowl.
4. In a large skillet heat up 1 tbsp. olive oil on medium-heat. Add your Italian sausage and stir occasionally while cooking the sausage. After about 5 or 8 minutes when the sausage has browned you can remove it.
5. Add spring onion, 1 tbsp. olive oil, and garlic and return the skillet to the heat and stir while cooking until onions become soft. This will take about 5 minutes. Add red peppers, zucchini, and Italian seasoning and stir continuously while cooking until the vegetables become soft. This will take about 5 minutes.
6. Stir feta cheese and spaghetti squash into the mixture of vegetables; stir while you cook until the cheese has melted. This will take about 3 minutes. Stir your sausage into the mixture of vegetables; season with lemon pepper and salt and sprinkle with parsley and tomatoes.

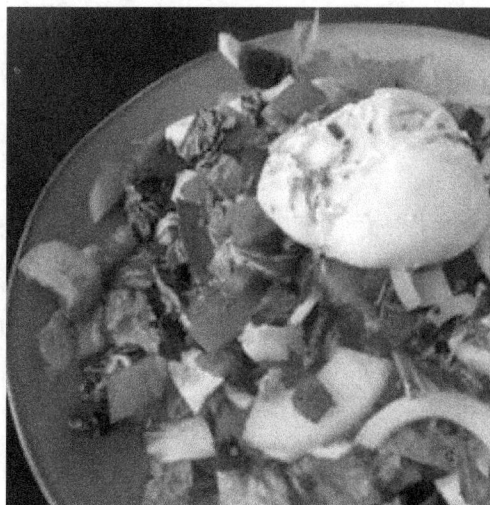

SaladeLyonnaise

(Total Time 50 | Servings 4)

Ingredients:

- 4 – eggs
- 1 Cup – Smoked bacon, chopped
- 2 Cloves – Garlic, finely chopped
- 1 Head – Romaine lettuce, chopped
- 2 – Roma tomatoes, sliced
- 2 Cups – Curly endive, chopped
- ½ Cup – Red wine vinegar
- 1 Cup – Extra virgin olive oil
- 1 Tsp. – White sugar
- 2 Tbsps. – Dijon mustard
- Salt and pepper to taste
- 2 Tbsps. – Herbs de Provence
- 1 Small = Onion, finely chopped

Directions:

1. In a large deep skillet lay out your bacon and cook on medium-high heat. Stir occasionally until bacon becomes browned. This will take about 10 minutes. Remove the bacon and lay the bacon out on a paper towel to drain.
2. Fill a large saucepan with water up to 2 to 3 inches and heat on high heat bringing it to a boil. Reduce to a medium-low heat and pour your vinegar into the simmering water. Crack and eggs and very gently slip them into the water and poach them until the egg whites are firm and yolks have become somewhat thick but not hard. This will take about 2 ½ to 3 minutes. Remove the poached eggs and dry them by dabbing them with a slotted spoon on a kitchen towel.
3. Using four plates divide your romaine lettuce and sprinkle with your garlic. Top all four salads with onion, tomatoes, poached egg and bacon.
4. In a separate bowl whisk red wine vinegar, olive oil, sugar, Dijon mustard, salt herbes de Provence, and pepper. Spoon the dressing over the four salads and serve.

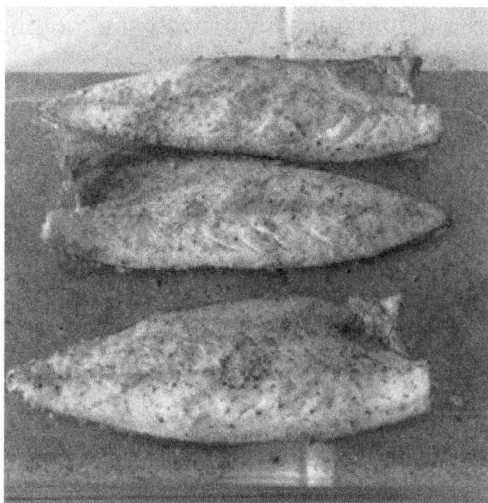

Broiled Spanish Mackerel
(Total Time 15 minutes | Servings 6 3 oz. fillets)

Ingredients:

- ¼ Cup – Olive oil
- 6 (3 oz.) – Fillets Spanish mackerel fillets
- Salt and ground black pepper to taste
- ½ Tsp. – Paprika
- 12 – Lemon, slices

Directions:
1. Preheat your oven on broil and move your bakers rack up about 6 inches from the top. Grease your baking dish lightly.
2. Rub olive oil over each mackerel fillets on both sides. Place them skin side down on your greased baking dish. Sprinkles the salt, pepper and paprika seasoning over the fillets. Place 2 lemon slices on top of each fillet.

3. Place the dish under the broiler to bake the fillets for 5 to 7 minutes until flaky.

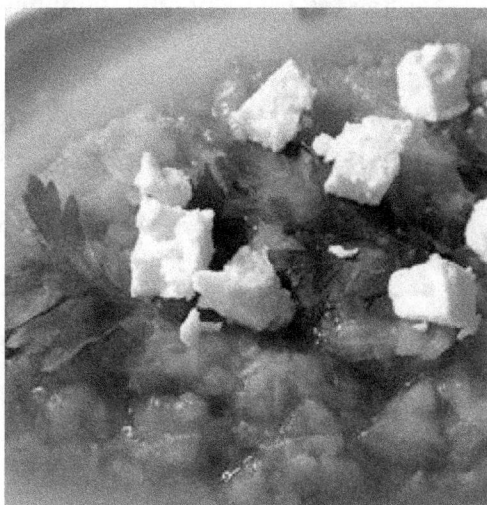

MelitzanosalataAgioritiki (Athenian Eggplant Salad)
(Total Time 2 hours | Servings 4 Cups)

Ingredients:

- 1 – Tomato, seeded and chopped
- 1 Large – Eggplant, washed
- 2 Tbsps. – Fresh parsley, chopped
- 1 Small – Onion, diced
- 2 Tbsps. – Distilled white vinegar
- 2 Tbsps. – Extra-virgin olive oil
- Salt to taste
- ½ Cup – Feta cheese crumbled

Directions:
1. Use an outdoor grill to preheat on medium-high heat.

2. Use a fork to poke holes in the eggplant and cook for about 15 minutes turning the eggplant often until the skin becomes charred and the inside tender.
3. After the eggplant has cooled enough remove the skin and dice the pulp. Place the eggplant, onion, tomato, olive oil, parsley, feta cheese and vinegar into a bowl. Mix the ingredients well and set in the refrigerator to cool for one hour. Remove from the refrigerator and salt before serving.

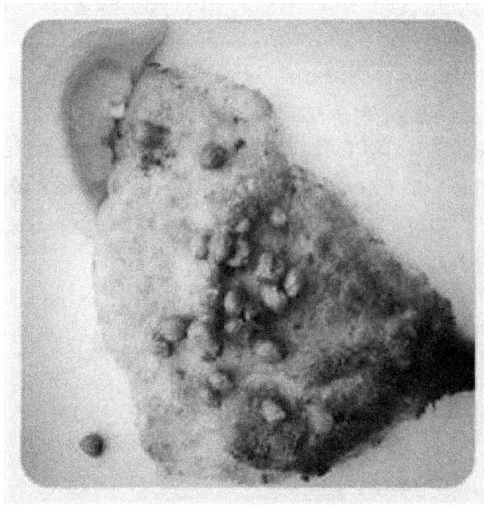

Lemon Caper Chicken
(Total Time 25 minutes | Servings 4)

Ingredients:

- ½ Tsp. – Ground black pepper
- 2 – Eggs
- 2 Tbsps. – Olive oil, or as needed.
- ¼ cup – Capers
- 1 ½ lbs. – Chicken breast halves, skinless, boneless, pounded ¾ inch thick and cut into pieces
- 2 – Lemons, cut into wedges

Directions:

1. Place black pepper and eggs in a bowl and beat together. In a separate shallow bowl place the bread crumbs.

2. In a large skillet heat olive oil on medium heat. Take the chicken pieces and dip them into the egg mixture and cover with bread crumbs. Remove excess bread crumbs from the chicken and drop the coated chicken in the hot oil. Fry the coated chicken for 5 to 8 minutes until a golden brown on both sides. Remove from the oil and place on a serving plate and drizzle the caper juice lightly over the fried chicken. Sprinkle capers over the chicken and place lemon wedges next to the chicken and serve.

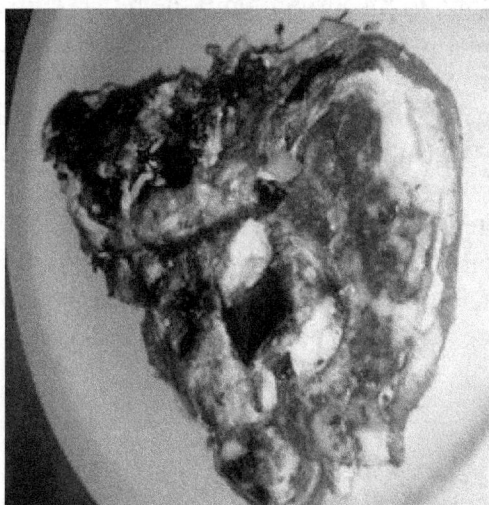

Portobello Pesto Egg Omelet
(Total Time 25 minutes | Servings 1 omelet)

Ingredients:

- 1 – Portobello mushroom cap, sliced
- 1 Tsp. – Olive oil
- 4 – Egg whites
- ¼ Cup – Red onion, chopped
- Salt and ground black pepper to taste
- 1 Tsp. – Water
- 1 Tsp. – Prepared pesto
- ¼ Cup – Low-fat mozzarella cheese, shredded

Directions:

1. In a skillet heat olive oil on medium heat. Cook the red onion and Portobello mushroom until the mushroom has become soft in the olive oil. This will take about 3 to 5 minutes.
2. Place the water and egg whites in a small bowl and whisk them together. Pour them in with the onion and mushroom mixture. Season the mixture with salt and pepper. Cook the mixture, stirring it occasionally until there is no more runny egg whites. This will take about 5 minutes. Sprinkle your mozzarella cheese over the top of the mixture and top that with your pesto. Fold the omelet over in half and cook until your cheese has melted. This will take about 2 to 3 minutes.

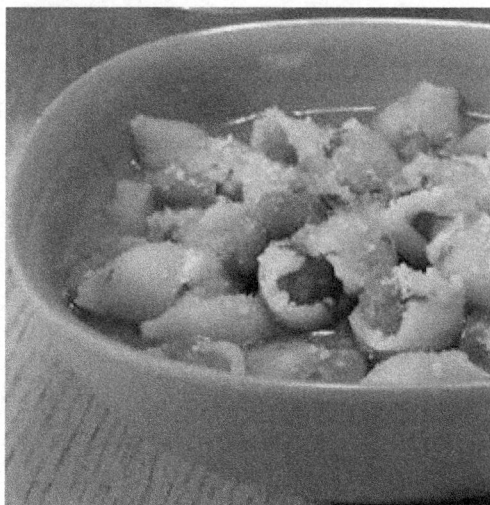

Classic Italian Pasta e Fagioli
(Total Time 1 hour| Servings 6)

Ingredients:

- 6 Cups – Cold water
- 2 Cups – Cranberry beans
- 2 Cups – Beef broth
- ½ Cup – White wine
- 3 Cloves – Garlic, crushed
- 4 ½ Cups – Chicken broth
- 2 Tbsps. – Fresh parsley, chopped
- 1 Tbsp. – Tomato paste
- 1/3 Cup – Parmesan cheese, grated
- 1 Pack (8 oz.) – Farfalle pasta
- 1 Tbsp. – Olive oil
- 2 Tbsps. - Parmesan cheese, grated

Directions:

1. Place water and cranberry beans in a large pot. Bring the mixture to a boil, turn off the heat and cover with a lid. Leave the pot on the burner for one hour to cool

2. Use a colander and drain your beans and return them to a large pot to cook. Add beef broth, wine and chicken broth. Bring the mixture to a boil and cover and let simmer for 30 minutes.

3. Place half of the beans in a food processor and puree them and add them back to the pot. Add the parsley, garlic, tomato paste, and farfalle pasta. Simmer uncovered for 25 to 30 minutes gently. When pasta becomes tender and soup is thick stir the parmesan cheese in and garnish with olive oil by drizzling it over top. Sprinkle the rest of the grated parmesan cheese over the top.

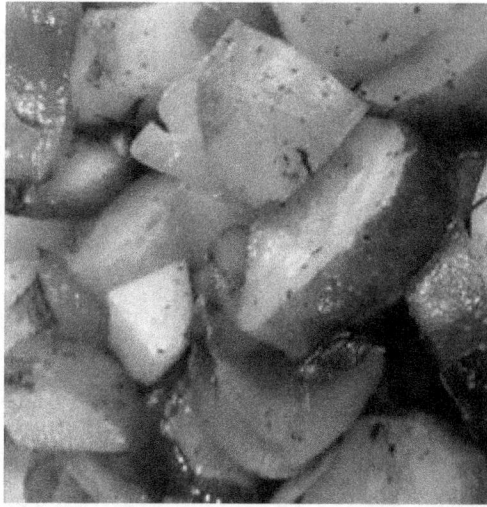

Mediterranean Roast Vegetables
(Total Time 1 hour and 30 minutes | Servings 4)

Ingredients:

- 2 – Red bell peppers, diced
- 6 Large – Potatoes, diced
- 1 – Zucchini, diced
- 1 – Fennel bulb, diced
- 6 Tbsps. – Olive oil
- 6 – Cloves garlic
- 2 Tsps. – Vegetable bouillon powder
- 2 Tsps. Salt
- ½ Cup – Balsamic vinegar
- ¼ Cup – Fresh rosemary, chopped

Directions:
1. Preheat your oven at 400 °F.

2. Place peppers, potatoes, zucchini, fennel, and garlic in a large baking dish. Take your olive oil and drizzle it evenly over the top of the vegetables. Sprinkle bouillon powder, salt and rosemary to coat the top of the vegetables.
3. Place the baking dish inside the oven to bake for about 1 hour, stirring occasionally until tender. Remove the vegetables from the oven and top with balsamic vinegar.

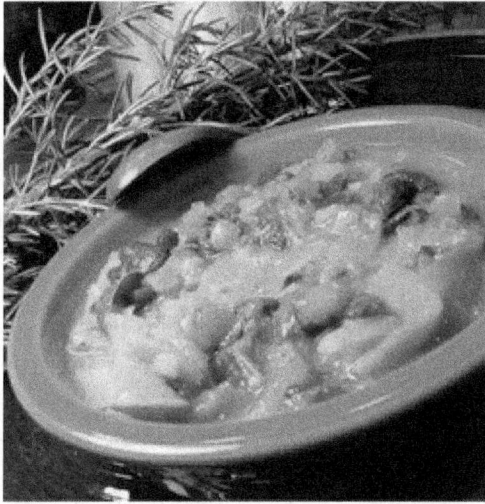

Italian Ribollita (Vegetable and Bread Soup)
(Total Time 10 hours | Servings 8)

Ingredients:

- 1 Large – Red onion, diced
- 1 Tbsp. – Olive oil
- 1 Stalk – Celery, diced
- 2 – Carrots, diced
- 10 (5 inch) – Zucchini, diced
- 4 – Potatoes, diced
- 1 Quart – hot water
- 1 – Leek, sliced
- 1 Head – Savoy cabbage, quartered, cored and shredded
- 1 Bunch – Swiss chard, chopped
- 2 Cans (15.5 oz.) – Cannellini beans, drained and rinsed
- 1 Bunch – Kale, shredded

- 3 Tbsps. – Tomato puree
- Salt and ground black pepper to taste
- 8 – Sliced day-old bread

Directions:

1. In a deep pan heat olive oil on medium-high. Stir the onion in and cook for about 5 minutes or until the onion becomes transparent. Mix the celery, carrots, zucchini, potatoes, and leek into the onion mix. Pour enough hot water in the pan to cover all the vegetables. Stir the Savoy cabbage, Swiss chard, and kale covering and simmering for 1 hour to reduce on medium heat.
2. Use the processor to blend 1 can of the beans and stir them into the vegetable mixture with the left over can of beans. Season with pepper and salt to taste. Reduce the heat and simmer on low for 20 minutes, stirring the mixture occasionally. Stir the tomato puree into the mix.
3. Using a casserole dish layer the vegetable mixture and bread slices. Cover the dish with plastic wrap and place in the refrigerator to cool for 8 hours.
4. Place the soup mixture into a pot and reheat on a medium heat.

Your Free Gift

I wanted to show my appreciation that you support my work so
I've put together a free gift for you.

Slowcooker Essentials Cookbook

http://thezenfactory.com/mediterranean_-diet-_free_book/

Just visit the link above to download it now.

I know you will love this gift.

Thanks!

Conclusion

The Mediterranean is well known for the amazing health factors that it contains. The people of the Mediterranean have less incidence of heart disease, lower risk factors for high blood pressure, cancer, diabetes and a wide array of other disorders. This is why the Mediterranean diet has health professionals stumped as to how the people live such a healthy life.

If you have been looking for one of the world's healthiest, most proven diet, the Mediterranean diet should be at the top of your list. It has been tried and true for many centuries. If you want to live a healthier lifestyle, this diet will amaze you. This is one of the few diets where you are able to enjoy flavorful food that has amazing quality and not feel guilty about it afterwards.

You will love the depth of flavors and the wide variety of foods that you can enjoy while you are eating this diet.

CPSIA information can be obtained
at www.ICGtesting.com
Printed in the USA
LVHW081257140319
610647LV00014B/173/P